A Doctor's Guide to

Living Well With DIABETES

(controlling sugar & preventing complications)

A Doctor's Guide to

Living Well With DIABETES

(controlling sugar & preventing complications)

Dr Prabhat Das

MD, PhD, FACP

Better Health with Dr Das Series

Disclaimer
This book is intended solely for educational and informational purposes. It is not meant to replace personal medical advice, diagnosis, or treatment. Although I am a licensed physician, reading this book does not establish a doctor–patient relationship. Each individual's health condition, medical history, and risk factors are unique. Any medical decision should be made in partnership with your own healthcare professional who understands your specific situation.
Medical science is continually advancing. New research and updated guidelines may lead to changes in recommendations over time.

Paperback ISBN: **978-1-971672-10-6**
eBook ISBN: **978-1-971672-11-3**

Typeset in font *Garamond* by *Indica Infomedia*, New Delhi, India
Printed in the United States of America

About the Author

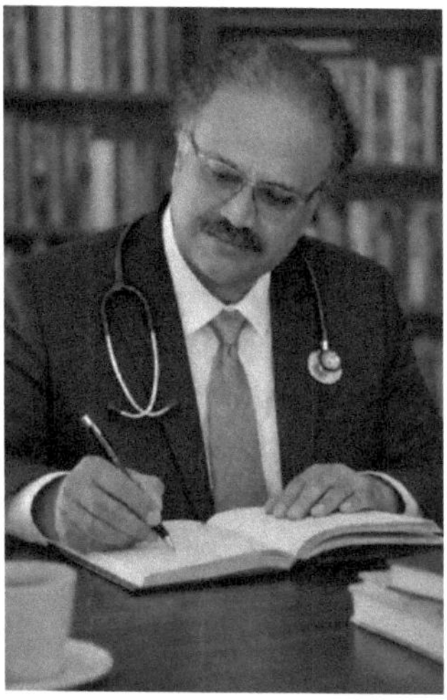

I am **Dr. Prabhat Das, MD, PhD, FACP**. My journey in medicine began in India, and for more than thirty five years I have had the privilege of practicing medicine in the United States. I am trained in **Internal Medicine, Pulmonary Diseases, and Critical Care**, and throughout these decades medicine has been far more than a career for me. It has been a lifelong calling rooted in learning, service, and deep respect for the people who place their trust in their physician.

Over the course of my medical career, I have cared for patients in many different settings. I have seen patients in my office for everyday health concerns, treated people in busy emergency rooms, managed complex illnesses in the hospital, and cared for the most critically ill patients in intensive care units. Thousands of patients have sat across from me during office visits. Many more have depended on careful decisions made during difficult and urgent moments in the hospital and ICU.

But medicine is not only about diagnoses, tests, and treatments. Every day I have listened to patients speak about their worries, their fears, their uncertainty, and often the many questions they hesitate to ask. Those conversations have taught me something profound. People want clear information, honest guidance, and reassurance they can trust. They want to understand their health so they can take better care of themselves and the people they love.

These experiences have shaped how I think about health, illness, prevention, and the deeply human side of healing.

Through the **"Better Health with Dr Das" series**, I hope to reach many individuals I may never meet personally in my office. Many people struggle quietly with health questions and confusing medical information. My goal in these books is simple. I want to explain important medical topics in a clear, practical, and reassuring way so that readers feel informed, confident, and empowered to make better decisions about their health. The information presented in these books is based on reliable scientific knowledge and decades of clinical experience.

If these books bring clarity to someone who feels confused, comfort to someone who feels worried, or practical help to someone trying to improve their health, then this effort will have been deeply worthwhile.

Helping people live healthier, better informed lives continues to be one of the greatest privileges and satisfactions of my professional life.

Table of Contents

Introduction

A Clear and Practical Path to Living Well with Diabetes

Over the years, I have met thousands of patients, in my office, in the hospital, and sometimes in urgent situations when they were at their most vulnerable.

Many of them had one thing in common.

They were not lacking effort. They were lacking clarity.

They had heard different things from different sources. Some advice was helpful. Some was confusing. Some created unnecessary fear. And in the middle of all this, they were trying their best to manage a condition that they did not fully understand.

That is the reason I wrote this book.

Not to overwhelm you with information, but to give you a clear, practical understanding of diabetes, in a way that makes sense in real life.

What this book is about

Diabetes is often reduced to numbers, blood sugar readings, A1c levels, lab reports.

These are important, but they are not the whole story.

Diabetes is about how your body handles energy. It is about how your daily habits influence your health. It is about protecting your heart, your brain, your kidneys, your eyes, and your overall well-being over time.

Most importantly, it is about how you live with it, day after day.

This book is designed to help you understand that clearly, without unnecessary complexity.

A simple and honest approach

In writing this book, I have followed one guiding principle.

Keep it simple, practical, and honest.

You will not find complicated medical language here. You will not find unrealistic promises or quick fixes.

Instead, you will find:

- clear explanations of how diabetes develops
- simple guidance on diet and lifestyle
- practical information about medications and insulin
- advice on preventing complications
- support for the emotional and social aspects of living with diabetes

Everything is explained in a way that you can understand and apply.

What I want you to feel while reading this

I do not want you to feel overwhelmed.

I want you to feel informed.

I do not want you to feel afraid.

I want you to feel prepared.

And most importantly, I want you to feel that you are in control of your health in a realistic and steady way.

A perspective from real-life practice

This book is not based only on theory.

It comes from years of clinical experience, seeing how patients actually live, what challenges they face, and what truly works over time.

I have seen patients struggle because they were confused.

I have also seen patients do remarkably well once they understood a few simple principles and followed them consistently.

That experience has shaped every chapter of this book.

There is no need for perfection

One of the most important ideas I want to share with you is this.

You do not need to be perfect to manage diabetes well.

In fact, trying to be perfect often leads to frustration.

What works is something much simpler.

A steady approach.

A few sensible habits, followed regularly.

Small improvements that continue over time.

That is how real progress happens.

This is a long-term journey

Diabetes is not a short-term condition.

It requires attention over time.

But that does not mean your life becomes limited or restricted.

With proper understanding and consistent care, you can continue to live fully.

You can work, travel, enjoy your family, and take part in all the activities that matter to you.

The goal of this book is not just control.

It is to help you live well.

How to use this book

You do not need to read this book in a hurry.

Take it one chapter at a time.

Focus on understanding the ideas.

Apply one or two changes at a time.

Return to important sections when needed.

This is not a book to read once and set aside.

It is a guide you can come back to.

A final thought before you begin

If you have recently been diagnosed, you may feel uncertain.

If you have been living with diabetes for years, you may feel tired or frustrated.

Wherever you are, I want you to remember one thing.

Diabetes is manageable.

Not in a dramatic or complicated way, but in a steady and practical way.

With understanding, consistency, and a balanced approach, you can take control of your health.

And that is what this book is here to help you do.

Chapter 1

Understanding Diabetes: Why It Matters More Than You May Realize

When you feel fine, but something important is changing

Over the years, many patients have come to my office for nothing more than a routine checkup. They sit down comfortably, smile, and say, "Doctor, I feel fine. I just came to make sure everything is all right."

Then a blood test tells a different story.

That moment often brings surprise, and sometimes disbelief. How can a person feel perfectly normal and still have diabetes?

This is one of the most important things to understand about this condition. Diabetes often begins quietly. It may not cause pain. It may not send a loud warning. It may not interrupt daily life in an obvious way. But slowly, silently, it can begin to affect the body.

That is why this subject matters so much. The goal is not to create fear. The goal is to create awareness, understanding, and the confidence to act early.

What diabetes really is

At its simplest, diabetes means that the level of glucose, or sugar, in the blood is higher than normal.

But that short definition does not tell the full story.

Glucose is not the enemy. It is one of the body's main sources of energy. Every cell depends on it. The brain, in particular, needs a steady supply of glucose to function properly. Muscles need it. Organs need it. Daily life depends on it.

For glucose to move from the bloodstream into the cells, the body needs insulin.

Insulin is a hormone made by the pancreas. You can think of it as a key. It helps unlock the door so glucose can enter the cells and be used as fuel.

In diabetes, this system does not work the way it should. The body may not make enough insulin. The cells may not respond to insulin properly. Sometimes both problems are present. When that happens, glucose stays in the blood instead of being used efficiently by the body.

That is where the trouble begins.

Why diabetes affects more than blood sugar

Many people think diabetes is simply a sugar problem. That is understandable, but it is incomplete.

High blood sugar is the starting point. Over time, however, the effects reach far beyond a lab number. Persistently high glucose can injure blood vessels, affect nerves, and place stress on important organs. This is why diabetes can lead to problems involving the heart, brain, kidneys, eyes, and feet.

In other words, diabetes is not important only because the blood sugar is high. It is important because of what that high blood sugar can quietly do to the body over the years.

At the same time, there is good news in that very same truth. When blood sugar comes under better control, the risk of many complications can be reduced. Better choices and better treatment truly matter. Improvement is not meaningless. It has real value.

Why this condition has become so common

Diabetes is now one of the most common chronic health problems in the world.

In the United States, millions of adults are living with diabetes, and many more have prediabetes without knowing it. The risk becomes greater with age, especially after 40, though younger adults and even children can be affected as well.

Why is diabetes so common now?

There is no single answer. Modern diet plays a role. Reduced physical activity plays a role. Excess weight, especially around the abdomen, is important. Family history and genetics are also powerful factors. In many people, several of these influences come together.

This is why diabetes has become so widespread. It is not the result of one simple mistake. It is usually the result of several forces acting together over time.

Diabetes is more than a number on a report

One of the most common mistakes people make is to reduce diabetes to a few numbers.

Patients often become focused on a fasting glucose value or an A1c result. These numbers are important, and we should pay attention to them. They help us diagnose the condition, monitor progress, and guide treatment.

But diabetes is not just a number.

It is about how well your body is functioning. It is about your energy, your circulation, your vision, your kidneys, your nerves, and your long-term health. Two people may have similar blood sugar readings and yet have very different outcomes depending on how consistently they care for themselves and how early the problem was recognized.

So yes, the numbers matter. But what matters even more is what those numbers mean in real life.

The fear people feel, and the truth they need

When patients first hear the word diabetes, I often see the same look in their eyes. There is uncertainty. Sometimes there is fear. Sometimes there is quiet disappointment. Many begin to imagine a future filled with restrictions, medicines, and complications.

Those feelings are understandable, but they are often shaped more by fear than by facts.

Over the years, I have also seen another side of the story. I have seen patients learn about their condition, make steady changes, follow treatment sensibly, and live very well for many years. They continue to work, travel, enjoy family life, celebrate holidays, and take part in the ordinary pleasures of life. Diabetes becomes a condition they manage, not a condition that controls them.

That is the truth patients need to hear early.

Diabetes is serious, but it is manageable. It deserves respect, not panic.

Why understanding must come before good control

One of the biggest barriers to good diabetes care is confusion.

When people do not understand what is happening inside their body, they often feel lost. They may try hard for a few days or a few weeks, but without clarity, motivation fades. Advice sounds like a list of rules rather than a meaningful plan.

The opposite is also true.

When a patient understands even the basic ideas, the whole experience changes. The condition becomes less mysterious. Decisions begin to make sense. Food choices feel less random. Treatment feels less like punishment and more like a tool.

That is why understanding comes first.

A patient who understands diabetes is in a much stronger position than a patient who is simply frightened by it.

A better way to think about diabetes

It may help to stop thinking of diabetes as a single problem and begin thinking of it as a condition that requires balance.

Balance in food.

Balance in movement.

Balance in daily routine.

Balance in medications, when they are needed.

Balance in expectations.

No single step solves everything. There is no magic food, no perfect pill, and no one habit that fixes the whole picture. But when several sensible steps come together, the body responds.

This is important, because many people either underestimate diabetes or overreact to it. Neither approach helps.

A balanced, informed, steady approach is far more powerful.

Small steps are not small when repeated every day

One of the reasons people feel overwhelmed is that they imagine they must change their entire life immediately.

That is rarely the best way.

The body usually changes gradually, and improvement also happens gradually. A slightly healthier breakfast. A daily walk. Taking medicine regularly. Sleeping better. Losing even a modest amount of weight. These may seem like small things. But repeated day after day, they become powerful.

This is true in medicine, and it is true in life.

Big results often come from small steps done consistently.

Looking ahead with the right mindset

Diabetes is not a short-term problem. It is a long-term condition, which means it responds best to long-term thinking.

That does not mean life becomes joyless or rigid. It means daily habits matter more than they may have mattered before. It means paying attention. It means making practical choices most of the time. It means accepting that good health is built slowly.

Most importantly, it means understanding that perfection is not required.

What matters is direction. What matters is staying engaged. What matters is continuing to move toward better control, better habits, and better health.

That is how people live well with diabetes.

Chapter 1 Summary

- Diabetes is a condition in which blood sugar remains higher than normal.
- It often begins quietly and may not cause obvious symptoms at first.
- Glucose is the body's fuel, and insulin helps move it into the cells.
- In diabetes, insulin is not sufficient, does not work properly, or both.
- High blood sugar over time can affect blood vessels, nerves, and major organs.
- Diabetes is common and becomes more likely with age, lifestyle factors, and family history.
- It is much more than a number on a lab report.
- With understanding and steady care, many people live well with diabetes.

Understanding Diabetes

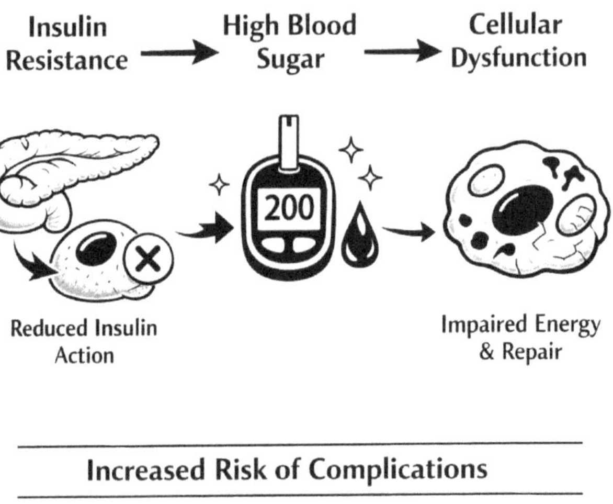

Action Plan

- Begin to think of diabetes as a manageable medical condition, not a personal failure.
- If you have risk factors, talk with your doctor about appropriate testing.
- Pay attention to your daily habits, especially food, activity, sleep, and weight.
- Do not wait for dramatic symptoms before taking your health seriously.
- Focus on small, realistic improvements rather than trying to change everything at once.
- Commit to learning your condition step by step.

Looking ahead

Now that we have a clear picture of what diabetes is and why it matters, the next step is to understand how it develops.

In the next chapter, we will look at the causes of diabetes, the role of insulin, the meaning of insulin resistance, and the different types of diabetes.

That discussion will help answer one of the most personal questions a patient can ask:

Why did this happen to me?

Chapter 2

How Diabetes Develops: Causes, Risk Factors, and Types

"Why did this happen to me?"

This is one of the first and most honest questions patients ask.

I have heard it many times, often with a quiet sense of worry, sometimes with guilt.

Let me say this clearly at the beginning.

Diabetes is rarely caused by one single reason.

It usually develops slowly, over years, due to a combination of factors. Some of these are within your control. Some are not.

Understanding this is important, because it replaces blame with clarity. And clarity allows you to move forward in a practical way.

How the body normally handles sugar

Every time you eat, especially foods containing carbohydrates such as rice, bread, fruits, or sweets, they are broken down into glucose.

This glucose enters the bloodstream and becomes available as fuel.

For the body to use this glucose, it must enter the cells. That process depends on insulin.

Insulin is produced by the pancreas. It acts like a key, allowing glucose to move from the blood into the cells.

In a healthy system, this works smoothly. Blood sugar rises after a meal and then gradually returns to normal as insulin does its job.

You eat, your blood sugar rises, insulin is released, and balance is restored.

What goes wrong in diabetes

In diabetes, this balance is disturbed.

There are two main problems:

- the body does not produce enough insulin
- the body's cells do not respond properly to insulin

The second problem is called insulin resistance.

In many people with type 2 diabetes, both of these problems are present.

At first, the body tries to compensate. The pancreas produces more insulin to keep blood sugar under control. For some time, this works.

But over the years, this system becomes less effective. The pancreas cannot keep up, and the cells remain resistant.

Gradually, blood sugar begins to rise.

Understanding insulin resistance

Insulin resistance is a key concept, and it is worth understanding in simple terms.

In this condition, the body's cells do not respond well to insulin.

Even though insulin is present, it is not working effectively.

To compensate, the pancreas produces more insulin.

This extra effort may continue for years, often without any symptoms. During this time, blood sugar may remain near normal, even though the underlying problem is developing.

Eventually, the pancreas becomes less able to keep up. At that point, blood sugar begins to rise, and diabetes becomes apparent.

What leads to insulin resistance

Insulin resistance does not occur randomly.

Several factors contribute to it:

- excess body weight, especially around the abdomen
- lack of physical activity

- genetic predisposition
- aging
- long-term dietary patterns

These factors do not act alone. In most patients, several are present together.

This is why diabetes develops differently in different people.

The role of the pancreas over time

The pancreas plays a central role in diabetes.

In the early stages, it works harder to compensate for insulin resistance by producing more insulin.

Over time, however, this increased demand cannot be sustained.

The ability of the pancreas to produce insulin gradually declines.

This is one of the reasons why diabetes may worsen over time and why medications may need to be adjusted.

It is not because the patient has failed.

It is because the body's capacity has changed.

The main types of diabetes

Understanding the types of diabetes helps make sense of treatment.

Type 1 diabetes

This is an autoimmune condition. The body's immune system

attacks the insulin-producing cells in the pancreas. As a result, little or no insulin is produced. Insulin is required for survival.

Type 2 diabetes

This is the most common type. It involves insulin resistance along with a gradual decline in insulin production. Lifestyle factors and genetics both play a role.

Prediabetes

Blood sugar levels are higher than normal but not high enough to be classified as diabetes. This stage is important because progression can often be slowed or prevented.

Gestational diabetes

This occurs during pregnancy. It usually improves after delivery but increases the risk of developing type 2 diabetes later.

Risk factors: what increases the likelihood

Some risk factors cannot be changed:

- age, especially after 40
- family history
- genetic background

Other risk factors can be influenced:

- excess body weight
- physical inactivity
- dietary habits

- poor sleep
- chronic stress

Having risk factors does not guarantee diabetes. But it increases the chance.

The encouraging part is that many of these factors can be improved.

Why diabetes appears differently in different people

You may wonder why one person develops diabetes earlier, while another does not, even with similar habits.

This is because people differ in how their bodies handle insulin.

Some develop insulin resistance more easily. Others have a reduced ability to produce insulin over time.

Fat distribution also matters. Weight around the abdomen is more strongly linked to insulin resistance than weight in other areas.

This is why diabetes is not a simple condition with a single cause.

Letting go of guilt

Many patients feel a sense of guilt after diagnosis.

"I should have taken better care of myself."

While lifestyle plays a role, it is only one part of the story.

Genetics, metabolism, and long-term patterns all contribute.

Guilt does not help.

Understanding does.

When you understand how diabetes develops, you can focus on what can be improved from this point forward.

A condition that develops gradually

One of the most important points to remember is this.

Diabetes usually develops slowly.

There is often a long period before diagnosis when blood sugar is rising gradually. During this time, there may be no symptoms at all.

This is why early testing is important.

It also means that improvement is possible, especially when changes are made early.

Chapter 2 Summary

- Diabetes develops gradually due to problems with insulin and insulin action
- Insulin helps glucose enter cells and provide energy
- Insulin resistance is a key factor in type 2 diabetes
- The pancreas may produce more insulin initially, then less over time
- The main types include type 1, type 2, prediabetes, and gestational diabetes
- Risk factors include age, genetics, weight, inactivity, and lifestyle

Etiologies of Diabetes

Understanding the Causes of Diabetes

Genetics

- Family History
- Genetic Mutations

Autoimmune Factors

- Type 1 Diabetes
- Latent Autoimmune Diabetes (LADA)

Pancreatic Disorders

- Pancreatitis
- Pancreatic Injury

Endocrine Disorders

- Cushing's Syndrome
- Acromegaly

Lifestyle Factors

- Sedentary Behavior
- Poor Diet
- Obesity

Medications & Chemicals

- Corticosteroids
- Certain Medications
- Toxins

Infections & Viruses

- Viral Infections
- Congenital Infections

Infections & Viruses

- Viral Infections
- Congenital Infections

- Diabetes has multiple causes, not a single reason
- Understanding the process helps guide better management

Action Plan

- Reflect on your personal risk factors without self-blame
- Begin making gradual improvements in daily habits
- Increase physical activity, even simple walking
- Work toward a healthy weight in a steady way
- Discuss screening and follow-up with your doctor
- Focus on understanding your condition rather than worrying about the past

Looking ahead

Now that you understand how diabetes develops, the next step is to recognize how it shows up in everyday life.

In the next chapter, we will discuss the signs and symptoms of diabetes, including the early clues that are often easy to miss.

Recognizing these signs can help you act at the right time.

Chapter 3

Recognizing Diabetes Early: Signs, Symptoms, and Silent Clues

The body often whispers before it speaks loudly

Many patients tell me something similar after they are diagnosed.

"Doctor, now that I think about it, there were signs. I just did not pay attention."

That is how diabetes often presents.

Not with dramatic symptoms, but with small, gradual changes that are easy to ignore. A little more tired than usual. A bit more thirsty. A few extra trips to the bathroom at night.

Life is busy. These changes do not seem important at first.

But sometimes, the body is quietly signaling that something is not quite right.

Learning to recognize these early clues can make a meaningful difference.

The classic symptoms

When blood sugar rises to a higher level, certain symptoms become more noticeable.

These include:

- increased thirst
- frequent urination
- increased hunger
- unexplained weight loss
- fatigue
- blurred vision

These symptoms are connected.

When blood sugar is high, the kidneys try to remove excess glucose through urine. This leads to more frequent urination. As fluid is lost, the body responds with increased thirst.

At the same time, the cells are not receiving glucose effectively. This leads to fatigue and increased hunger.

Subtle signs that are easy to miss

In many people, especially those with type 2 diabetes, symptoms are mild or vague.

You may notice:

- persistent tiredness
- reduced concentration
- mild headaches
- frequent infections
- slow healing of small cuts
- dry or itchy skin

These symptoms are often attributed to stress, aging, or a busy lifestyle.

Because of this, diabetes can remain undiagnosed for a long time.

Fatigue that feels different

Fatigue in diabetes is not just ordinary tiredness.

It is a sense of low energy that does not improve much with rest.

The reason is simple. The body is not using glucose properly. Even though there is enough sugar in the blood, the cells are not getting the energy they need.

This can leave you feeling tired without a clear reason.

Thirst and frequent urination

These two symptoms often occur together and are important warning signs.

High blood sugar leads to increased glucose in the urine. This draws water out of the body.

As a result:

- you urinate more often
- your body loses fluid
- you feel more thirsty

Some patients notice waking up several times at night to urinate. This should not be ignored, especially if it is new.

Changes in vision

High blood sugar can affect the lens of the eye.

You may notice:

- blurred vision
- difficulty focusing
- vision that seems to change from day to day

In early stages, these changes are often temporary and improve with better blood sugar control.

Weight changes

Unexplained weight loss can be an early sign, particularly when diabetes is more advanced.

When the body cannot use glucose effectively, it begins to break down fat and muscle for energy.

On the other hand, some people may gain weight over time due to insulin resistance and lifestyle factors.

Both patterns are important to recognize.

Infections and slow healing

Another clue is an increased tendency toward infections.

Patients may experience:

- frequent urinary infections
- skin infections
- gum problems
- fungal infections

Cuts and wounds may also take longer to heal.

High blood sugar affects the body's ability to fight infection and repair tissue.

When there are no symptoms at all

One of the most important points in this chapter is this.

Many people with diabetes have no symptoms in the early stages.

They feel completely normal.

This is why screening is important, especially if you have risk factors.

Waiting for symptoms is not always a safe approach.

Why early recognition matters

Detecting diabetes early can change its course.

When identified early:

- lifestyle changes are more effective
- blood sugar is easier to control
- the risk of complications is lower

When diagnosis is delayed, high blood sugar continues to affect the body quietly.

Paying attention without becoming anxious

There is a balance to maintain.

You do not need to worry about every small symptom. But it is important to notice changes that persist or do not have a clear explanation.

A calm and attentive approach is more helpful than ignoring symptoms or becoming overly anxious.

Chapter 3 Summary

- Diabetes often develops with subtle or unnoticed symptoms
- Common symptoms include thirst, frequent urination, fatigue, and blurred vision
- Early signs may be mild and easily overlooked
- Fatigue occurs because the body is not using glucose

Signs and Symptoms of Diabetes

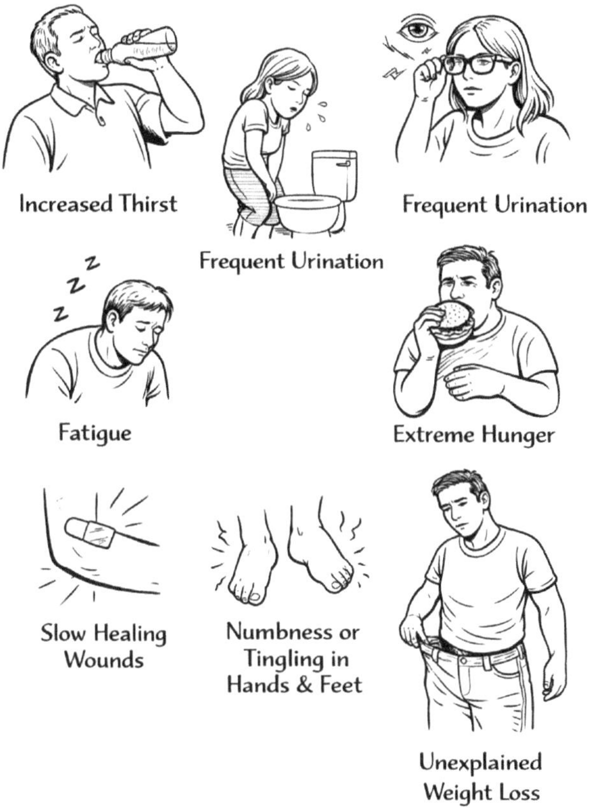

effectively

- Vision changes may occur early and can improve with better control
- Infections and slow healing are important clues
- Some people have no symptoms in early stages
- Early detection improves outcomes

Action Plan

- pay attention to persistent symptoms such as fatigue or increased thirst
- do not ignore frequent infections or slow healing
- consider regular screening if you have risk factors
- keep a simple record of ongoing symptoms
- discuss concerns with your doctor early
- stay aware without becoming anxious

Looking ahead

Recognizing symptoms is an important step.

In the next chapter, we will discuss how diabetes is diagnosed and monitored, and what the different tests mean.

This will help you move from uncertainty to clarity.

Chapter 4

Diagnosis and Monitoring: Understanding Your Numbers with Confidence

From uncertainty to clarity

For many patients, this stage brings mixed emotions.

Some feel surprised. Others feel worried. A few are unsure whether the diagnosis is truly correct.

I often tell my patients something simple.

A diagnosis does not create the disease. It reveals it.

Once you have clarity, you can take the right steps. Without it, diabetes can continue quietly without direction.

This chapter is about making that clarity simple, practical, and useful in your daily life.

How diabetes is diagnosed

Diabetes is diagnosed using well-established blood tests. These tests are simple, reliable, and widely used.

The most common ones include:

Fasting blood glucose

This test is done after an overnight fast. It shows how your body manages blood sugar when you have not eaten.

Hemoglobin A1c (HbA1c)

This test reflects your average blood sugar over the past two to three months. It gives a broader picture than a single reading.

Oral glucose tolerance test (OGTT)

After drinking a glucose solution, blood sugar is measured over time to see how your body processes sugar.

Random blood glucose

This can be measured at any time, especially when symptoms are present.

Each of these tests provides useful information. Together, they help confirm the diagnosis.

Making sense of the numbers

Patients often feel confused when they see their results.

"What do these numbers actually mean?"

You do not need to remember exact cutoffs.

Think of it in a simple way:

- normal values suggest your body is handling glucose well
- slightly elevated values suggest prediabetes
- higher values confirm diabetes

The A1c is especially helpful because it reflects long-term control.

It is not influenced by a single meal. It shows the average over time.

Why confirmation is sometimes needed

In some cases, a single abnormal test is not enough.

Your doctor may repeat the test or use another test for confirmation.

This is done to ensure accuracy.

Temporary factors such as illness, stress, or certain medications can affect blood sugar.

A confirmed diagnosis allows you to move forward with confidence.

Monitoring after diagnosis

Once diabetes is diagnosed, monitoring becomes an important part of care.

Monitoring helps answer key questions:

- Is the treatment working?
- Are your levels improving?

- Do adjustments need to be made?

There are two main approaches.

Home blood glucose monitoring

A small device is used to check blood sugar from a fingerstick. It provides immediate results.

Continuous glucose monitoring (CGM)

A small sensor placed under the skin measures glucose throughout the day and night. It shows patterns and trends.

Both methods are useful. The choice depends on your situation.

Understanding daily variation

Many patients feel concerned when they see changes in their readings.

It is important to know that some variation is normal.

Blood sugar levels are influenced by:

- food
- physical activity
- stress
- sleep
- medications

Instead of focusing on a single number, look for patterns.

Are your readings generally improving? Are certain times of day consistently higher?

These patterns are much more useful.

The role of A1c in long-term care

Daily readings show what is happening now.

The A1c shows what has been happening over the past few months.

It answers an important question.

How well has your blood sugar been controlled over time?

This helps guide long-term treatment decisions.

How often should testing be done

Testing frequency varies from person to person.

For those at risk, periodic screening is enough.

For those with diabetes:

- A1c is usually checked every few months
- home monitoring may be daily or periodic

Your doctor will guide you based on your needs.

Becoming an active participant

One of the most encouraging changes I see is when patients begin to understand their numbers.

Instead of feeling anxious, they begin to use the information.

They start asking:

- what is affecting my readings?
- what can I improve?

This shift makes a significant difference.

Avoiding common misunderstandings

A few important points to remember:

- one normal reading does not rule out diabetes
- mildly elevated values should not be ignored
- very tight control is not necessary for everyone

Treatment should always be individualized.

Clarity builds confidence

When you understand your tests and numbers, something important happens.

You feel more confident.

The numbers stop being confusing. They begin to guide you.

Chapter 4 Summary

- Diabetes is diagnosed using blood tests such as fasting glucose and A1c
- A1c reflects average blood sugar over two to three months

- Diagnosis may require confirmation
- Monitoring helps guide treatment
- Blood sugar varies based on multiple factors
- Patterns are more important than single readings
- Understanding your numbers improves confidence

Action Plan

- learn the basic meaning of your test results
- follow recommended testing schedules
- keep a simple record of your readings
- look for patterns rather than isolated values
- discuss your results with your doctor
- stay engaged in your care

Looking ahead

Now that you understand diagnosis and monitoring, the next step is to look at what these numbers mean for your body.

In the next chapter, we will explore how diabetes affects different organs and why long-term control is so important.

Chapter 5

How Diabetes Affects the Body: What Is Happening Inside

Looking beyond the report

By now, you understand how diabetes is diagnosed and how blood sugar is measured.

But an important question remains.

What do these numbers actually mean for your body?

I often tell my patients that numbers are only signals. They point to something deeper. What truly matters is what is happening inside the body over time.

When you understand this, your focus shifts. You are no longer just checking a value. You are protecting your organs, your energy, and your long-term health.

Why high blood sugar causes harm

Glucose is essential for life. Every cell depends on it.

But when glucose remains elevated for long periods, it begins to create problems.

Over time, high blood sugar can:

- damage the inner lining of blood vessels
- affect nerve function
- interfere with normal cellular activity
- increase inflammation in the body

These changes happen slowly. In the early stages, you may not feel anything at all.

That is why diabetes is often described as a silent condition.

Blood vessels at the center

To understand diabetes, it helps to understand blood vessels.

Blood vessels carry oxygen and nutrients to every part of the body.

When these vessels are affected, multiple organs are affected.

There are two main types involved:

Large blood vessels

These supply the heart and brain. Damage here increases the risk of heart disease and stroke.

Small blood vessels

These supply delicate tissues such as the eyes, kidneys, and nerves. Damage here leads to many common complications of diabetes.

This is why diabetes has such a wide impact.

Nerves and sensation

Nerves are especially sensitive to high blood sugar.

Over time, nerve damage can develop.

Patients may notice:

- tingling or burning sensations
- numbness
- sharp or shooting pain

Loss of sensation is particularly important.

When feeling is reduced, small injuries may go unnoticed. A minor cut or blister can become a larger problem if it is not treated.

Short-term and long-term effects

It is helpful to think about diabetes in two ways.

Short-term effects

These include fatigue, increased thirst, and frequent urination. They are often reversible with better blood sugar control.

Long-term effects

These involve gradual damage to blood vessels and organs over many years.

The important point is this.

Long-term complications are not inevitable. They depend largely on how diabetes is managed.

The power of steady control

One of the most encouraging truths in diabetes care is that improvement matters.

When blood sugar is kept within a reasonable range:

- damage to blood vessels slows
- nerve injury is reduced
- the risk of complications decreases

Even moderate improvement can make a meaningful difference.

This is why consistency is more important than perfection.

Inflammation and internal balance

High blood sugar creates a state of low-level inflammation in the body.

This contributes to damage in blood vessels and tissues.

Lifestyle factors such as poor diet, inactivity, and excess weight can make this worse.

On the other hand, healthy habits help restore balance and support healing.

The body's ability to improve

The body has a remarkable ability to respond when conditions improve.

When blood sugar is better controlled:

- cells function more efficiently
- inflammation may decrease
- energy levels often improve

While advanced damage may not always be reversible, early changes can be slowed or improved.

Diabetes does not decide your future

A diagnosis of diabetes does not determine what will happen next.

Outcomes vary widely.

They depend on:

- how well blood sugar is controlled
- daily habits
- timely medical care
- regular follow-up

Two people with the same diagnosis can have very different results.

Your daily actions matter.

A practical way to think about it

Instead of focusing only on disease, think in terms of protection.

Each healthy choice helps protect your blood vessels, nerves, and organs.

Each step contributes to your long-term health.

Small steps, lasting results

Many patients feel overwhelmed when thinking about long-term complications.

I suggest a simpler approach.

Focus on small, consistent actions:

- a healthier meal
- a daily walk
- taking medications regularly
- monitoring blood sugar

These steps may seem simple, but over time, they have a powerful effect.

Chapter 5 Summary

- High blood sugar over time damages blood vessels,

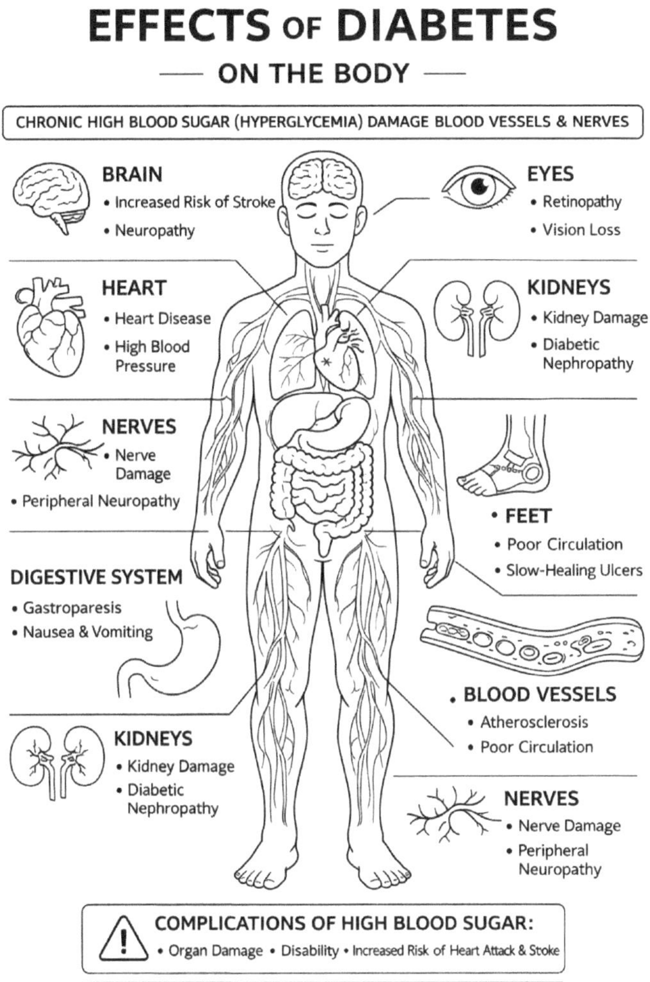
EFFECTS OF DIABETES
ON THE BODY
CHRONIC HIGH BLOOD SUGAR (HYPERGLYCEMIA) DAMAGE BLOOD VESSELS & NERVES
BRAIN
• Increased Risk of Stroke
• Neuropathy
EYES
• Retinopathy
• Vision Loss
HEART
• Heart Disease
• High Blood Pressure
KIDNEYS
• Kidney Damage
• Diabetic Nephropathy
NERVES
• Nerve Damage
• Peripheral Neuropathy
• FEET
• Poor Circulation
• Slow-Healing Ulcers
DIGESTIVE SYSTEM
• Gastroparesis
• Nausea & Vomiting
BLOOD VESSELS
• Atherosclerosis
• Poor Circulation
KIDNEYS
• Kidney Damage
• Diabetic Nephropathy
NERVES
• Nerve Damage
• Peripheral Neuropathy
COMPLICATIONS OF HIGH BLOOD SUGAR:
• Organ Damage • Disability • Increased Risk of Heart Attack & Stoke

nerves, and organs

- Both large and small blood vessels are affected
- Nerve damage can reduce sensation and increase risk of injury
- Short-term symptoms are often reversible
- Long-term complications depend on management
- Steady control reduces risk
- Healthy habits support the body's natural balance
- Small, consistent actions lead to better outcomes

Action Plan

- focus on steady blood sugar control
- pay attention to early changes such as numbness or vision issues
- follow your treatment plan consistently
- build simple, daily habits
- stay informed about how diabetes affects your body
- think in terms of protecting your long-term health

Looking ahead

Now that you understand how diabetes affects the body as a whole, the next step is to look at specific organs in more detail.

In the next chapter, we will focus on how diabetes affects the heart, brain, and blood vessels, and how you can protect them.

Chapter 6

Diabetes and the Heart, Brain, and Blood Vessels

Why this matters more than most people realize

When people think about diabetes, they often think only about blood sugar.

But in day-to-day practice, one of our biggest concerns is something else.

The heart and the blood vessels.

Many of the serious complications of diabetes are not caused directly by high sugar alone, but by the effect it has over time on circulation. This is why heart disease and stroke are so closely linked with diabetes.

This may sound concerning, but there is an important and reassuring point.

Much of this risk can be reduced with steady and sensible care.

What happens to blood vessels over time

Blood vessels are lined with a delicate inner surface. This lining helps maintain smooth blood flow.

When blood sugar remains high over time, this lining is affected.

Gradually:

- the vessels become less flexible
- the inner surface becomes less healthy
- narrowing may begin

Over time, this process can reduce blood flow.

This is often referred to as hardening of the arteries.

Why the heart is affected

The heart depends on a continuous supply of blood through the coronary arteries.

When these arteries become narrowed or blocked, the heart muscle does not receive enough oxygen.

This can lead to:

- chest discomfort or pressure
- reduced ability to tolerate activity
- heart attacks

People with diabetes are at higher risk for two main reasons.

First, the blood vessels are more vulnerable.

Second, other risk factors are often present at the same time.

The role of other risk factors

Diabetes rarely occurs alone.

Many patients also have:

- high blood pressure
- abnormal cholesterol levels
- excess body weight

These conditions work together and increase the strain on blood vessels.

When combined, they significantly increase the risk of heart disease.

Diabetes and stroke

The same process that affects the heart can also affect the brain.

If blood flow to part of the brain is reduced or blocked, a stroke can occur.

This may lead to:

- weakness on one side of the body
- difficulty speaking
- problems with balance
- changes in thinking

Some effects may improve with time, but others can be long-lasting.

Prevention is therefore very important.

Circulation in the legs

Blood flow to the legs can also be affected.

Patients may notice:

- pain or discomfort while walking
- slower healing of wounds
- increased risk of infections

Reduced circulation, combined with nerve damage, increases the risk of foot problems.

Symptoms are not always obvious

One of the challenges in diabetes is that symptoms may not always be typical.

Heart problems may not always present as clear chest pain.

Instead, patients may experience:

- shortness of breath
- unusual fatigue
- mild discomfort in the chest, neck, or jaw

Similarly, early signs of stroke may be subtle.

Any sudden change in speech, vision, strength, or coordination should be taken seriously.

The importance of blood pressure and cholesterol

Controlling blood sugar alone is not enough.

Blood pressure and cholesterol play a major role in protecting the heart and brain.

Managing these factors reduces risk significantly.

This often involves:

- lifestyle changes
- medications when needed
- regular monitoring

Protecting your heart and brain

There are clear and practical steps that help reduce risk:

- maintaining reasonable blood sugar control
- staying physically active
- eating a balanced diet
- maintaining a healthy weight
- controlling blood pressure and cholesterol
- avoiding smoking

Each of these contributes to better cardiovascular health.

Small steps that add up

Patients sometimes feel that these changes are too many.

The key is to begin with small steps.

A daily walk. A slightly healthier meal. Taking medications regularly.

These actions may seem modest, but over time, they have a meaningful effect.

The value of regular follow-up

Routine medical care is important.

Regular visits allow your doctor to:

- monitor risk factors
- adjust treatment
- detect early changes

Preventing complications is always easier than treating them later.

A realistic and reassuring perspective

It is important to keep this in balance.

Diabetes increases risk, but it does not guarantee complications.

Many patients maintain good heart and brain health for years.

The difference lies in awareness, consistency, and steady care.

Chapter 6 Summary

- Diabetes increases the risk of heart disease and stroke
- High blood sugar affects the inner lining of blood vessels
- Blood pressure and cholesterol often add to the risk
- Circulation problems can affect the legs
- Symptoms may be subtle or atypical
- Managing multiple risk factors is essential
- Healthy habits significantly reduce risk
- Regular follow-up supports prevention

Action Plan

- monitor blood pressure and cholesterol regularly
- stay physically active
- follow a heart-healthy diet
- take medications as prescribed
- avoid smoking
- watch for warning signs such as shortness of breath or weakness
- maintain regular medical visits

Looking ahead

In this chapter, we focused on the larger blood vessels and their effect on the heart and brain.

In the next chapter, we will look at smaller blood vessels and how diabetes affects the eyes, kidneys, and nerves.

Understanding this will help you take practical steps to protect these vital organs.

Chapter 7

Diabetes and the Eyes, Kidneys, and Nerves: Protecting the Silent Systems

Problems you may not feel until late

In the last chapter, we focused on the heart and large blood vessels.

Now we turn to something more subtle, and in many ways, more dangerous.

Damage to small blood vessels.

These vessels are delicate. They supply the eyes, kidneys, and nerves. When they are affected, the changes are often slow and silent.

Many patients feel completely normal during the early stages.

That is what makes this important.

By the time symptoms appear, the problem may already be

advanced.

The goal, therefore, is not just treatment. The goal is early awareness and protection.

How small vessel damage develops

The body contains a network of very fine blood vessels that nourish sensitive tissues.

High blood sugar affects these vessels over time.

Gradually:

- the vessel walls become less healthy
- blood flow becomes less efficient
- tissues receive less oxygen and nutrients

This process is slow, but persistent.

It leads to damage in specific organs that depend on these small vessels.

Diabetes and the eyes

The retina is a delicate layer at the back of the eye that allows you to see clearly.

It depends on a fine network of small blood vessels.

When these vessels are affected, a condition called diabetic retinopathy develops.

In the early stages, there are usually no symptoms.

As the condition progresses, patients may notice:

- blurred or fluctuating vision
- difficulty reading
- dark spots or floaters
- reduced night vision

If not detected early, it can lead to significant vision loss.

Here is the reassuring part.

Regular eye examinations can detect early changes before you notice anything. With timely care, many serious problems can be prevented.

Diabetes and the kidneys

The kidneys act as filters for the blood.

They remove waste and maintain the body's internal balance.

Inside the kidneys are tiny filtering units that are very sensitive to blood sugar levels.

When these are affected, diabetic kidney disease develops.

In the early stages, there are no symptoms.

Later, patients may notice:

- swelling in the feet or ankles
- changes in urination
- fatigue

- rising blood pressure

Routine blood and urine tests can detect early changes long before symptoms appear.

Early treatment can slow or even prevent further damage.

Diabetes and the nerves

Nerve damage, known as diabetic neuropathy, is common and important.

It most often affects the feet and legs.

Patients may experience:

- tingling
- burning sensation
- numbness
- sharp or shooting pain

Loss of sensation is particularly concerning.

A small injury may go unnoticed. Over time, this can lead to infection or more serious problems.

This is why daily foot care becomes so important in diabetes.

Why these complications are often silent

One of the most important points to understand is this.

These complications develop quietly.

There is often no pain in the early stages. No warning that something is changing.

That is why waiting for symptoms is not a safe approach.

Regular screening is essential.

The importance of routine screening

Simple tests can detect early changes.

These include:

- regular eye examinations
- blood tests for kidney function
- urine tests for protein
- foot examinations

These tests are not complicated, but they are very powerful.

They allow early detection and early action.

The role of blood sugar and overall control

Across all these complications, one principle remains consistent.

Better control reduces risk.

This includes:

- maintaining reasonable blood sugar levels
- controlling blood pressure

- managing cholesterol

These factors work together to protect your organs.

What you can do every day

Patients often ask, “What can I do to protect myself?”

The answer lies in simple, consistent habits:

- keep blood sugar under steady control
- monitor your health regularly
- stay physically active
- follow a balanced diet
- avoid smoking
- attend regular medical checkups

These steps are simple, but they are effective.

A reassuring perspective

It is natural to feel concerned when you hear about complications.

But they are not inevitable.

Many patients maintain good vision, healthy kidneys, and normal nerve function for many years.

The difference lies in awareness, consistency, and early action.

Chapter 7 Summary

- Diabetes affects small blood vessels supplying eyes, kidneys, and nerves
- Eye disease may develop without early symptoms
- Kidney disease is often silent in early stages
- Nerve damage can cause pain or loss of sensation
- Routine screening is essential for early detection
- Blood sugar, blood pressure, and cholesterol control reduce risk
- Daily habits play an important role
- Early action can prevent serious complications

Action Plan

- schedule regular eye examinations
- follow recommended kidney testing
- check your feet daily
- maintain steady blood sugar control
- monitor blood pressure regularly
- attend routine follow-up visits

Looking ahead

Now that you understand how diabetes affects important organs, we turn to something even more practical.

In the next chapter, we will focus on everyday care, your feet, skin, teeth, and protection from infections.

These are areas where small daily attention can prevent larger problems.

Chapter 8

Daily Care That Protects You: Feet, Skin, Teeth, and Infections

Where small details make a big difference

Up to this point, we have discussed how diabetes affects major organs.

Now we come to something more practical. The small, everyday details.

A dry patch of skin. A small cut on the foot. Bleeding gums. A minor infection that lingers longer than expected.

In most people, these are minor issues.

In diabetes, they deserve more attention.

Not because they are dangerous by themselves, but because they can become serious if they are ignored.

In my practice, I have seen both sides. A small problem caught early and treated easily. And the same problem, overlooked for weeks, becoming much more difficult to manage.

The difference is often simple awareness.

Why the feet need special attention

Foot care is one of the most important parts of daily diabetes management.

There are two main reasons.

First, nerve damage can reduce sensation. You may not feel pain from a small injury.

Second, circulation may be reduced, which slows healing.

When these two factors come together, even a small problem can worsen if it is not noticed early.

Common foot problems

Patients with diabetes may develop:

- dry or cracked skin
- calluses or corns
- blisters from tight shoes
- small cuts or ulcers
- infections

Because sensation may be reduced, these may not cause

discomfort.

That is why regular inspection is essential.

A simple daily foot routine

Foot care does not need to be complicated.

A few simple steps make a significant difference:

- check your feet daily, including between the toes
- wash your feet with lukewarm water
- dry them gently, especially between the toes
- apply moisturizer to prevent dryness, but not between the toes
- trim nails carefully
- wear comfortable, well-fitting shoes
- avoid walking barefoot

This routine takes only a few minutes, but it can prevent major problems.

Caring for your skin

The skin is your body's first line of protection.

In diabetes, the skin may become dry and more prone to irritation and infection.

You may notice:

- dryness or itching
- minor rashes
- small cracks in the skin

Keeping the skin clean and moisturized helps maintain its protective function.

Treating small problems early

Even a small cut or scratch should be taken seriously.

Clean it gently, keep it dry, and observe it closely.

Watch for signs such as:

- redness
- swelling
- warmth
- discharge

If a wound is not healing or appears to worsen, seek medical advice early.

A small problem is much easier to treat at the beginning.

Oral health and diabetes

Oral health is often overlooked, but it is closely linked with diabetes.

High blood sugar increases the risk of gum disease and infections.

You may notice:

- bleeding gums
- swelling or tenderness
- bad breath
- loosening of teeth

Good oral hygiene is essential.

- brush regularly
- floss daily
- visit your dentist routinely

Healthy gums are an important part of overall health.

Why infections are more common

People with diabetes are more prone to infections.

High blood sugar can:

- weaken the body's natural defense system
- allow bacteria and fungi to grow more easily

Common infections include:

- skin infections
- urinary infections
- fungal infections
- dental infections

These infections may take longer to heal if blood sugar is not well controlled.

Recognizing warning signs

It is important to act early.

Seek medical advice if you notice:

- redness or swelling
- increasing pain
- discharge from a wound
- fever or general illness
- a cut that is not healing

Early treatment prevents complications.

Building simple daily habits

Patients sometimes feel that diabetes care involves too many steps.

The key is to keep it simple and consistent.

Focus on a few habits:

- check your feet
- care for your skin
- maintain oral hygiene
- follow your treatment plan

Over time, these habits become part of your routine.

Prevention is always easier

One of the most reassuring aspects of diabetes care is this.

Many complications can be prevented.

Daily attention to small details can avoid larger problems later.

Chapter 8 Summary

- Diabetes affects daily health, including feet, skin, and oral health
- Reduced sensation and circulation increase the risk of foot problems
- Daily foot inspection is essential
- Skin may become dry and prone to infection
- Gum disease is more common in diabetes
- Infections occur more easily and may heal slowly
- Early attention prevents complications
- Simple daily habits are highly effective

Action Plan

- inspect your feet daily
- keep your skin clean and moisturized

- maintain good oral hygiene
- wear proper footwear and avoid walking barefoot
- treat small wounds early
- seek medical advice for signs of infection
- build a consistent daily routine

Looking ahead

So far, we have focused on problems that develop gradually.

In the next chapter, we will discuss situations that can develop quickly and need immediate attention.

We will talk about low blood sugar, diabetic ketoacidosis, and severe high blood sugar.

Understanding these will help you act quickly and confidently when needed.

Chapter 9

Diabetes Emergencies: When You Must Act Quickly

When control changes suddenly

Most of diabetes is slow and steady.

But there are times when things change quickly.

I have seen patients who were doing reasonably well suddenly feel shaky, confused, or very unwell within a short period. In some cases, a family member notices the change before the patient does.

These situations are called diabetes emergencies.

The purpose of this chapter is not to create fear.

It is to help you recognize these situations early and respond calmly and correctly.

Hypoglycemia: when blood sugar drops too low

Hypoglycemia, or low blood sugar, is one of the most common urgent problems in diabetes.

It is more likely in people taking insulin or certain oral medications.

It may occur when:

- a meal is delayed or missed
- medication dose is higher than needed
- physical activity increases without adjustment
- alcohol is taken without enough food

Early warning signs of low blood sugar

Low blood sugar often develops quickly.

Early symptoms include:

- sweating
- shakiness
- hunger
- anxiety or nervousness
- palpitations

If not treated, it may progress to:

- confusion
- difficulty speaking

- blurred vision
- weakness

In severe cases, it can lead to unconsciousness or seizures.

What to do immediately

The most important rule is simple.

Act without delay.

Take a fast-acting source of glucose such as:

- glucose tablets
- fruit juice
- regular soda

Wait about 15 minutes and reassess your symptoms. If needed, repeat.

Once you feel better, take a small snack or meal to prevent the blood sugar from dropping again.

Preventing low blood sugar

Prevention is always better than treatment.

- eat meals on time
- monitor blood sugar regularly
- adjust medication when needed
- plan for physical activity

- be cautious with alcohol

Over time, you will learn how your body responds.

Diabetic ketoacidosis (DKA)

DKA is a serious condition that requires urgent attention.

It occurs when the body does not have enough insulin.

Without insulin, glucose cannot enter the cells. The body then begins to break down fat for energy, producing substances called ketones. These make the blood acidic.

This condition can worsen quickly.

Warning signs of DKA

Symptoms may include:

- nausea and vomiting
- abdominal pain
- deep or rapid breathing
- fruity odor of the breath
- severe fatigue
- confusion

DKA is more common in type 1 diabetes but can occur in type 2 diabetes during illness or stress.

When urgent care is needed

DKA cannot be managed at home.

It requires hospital treatment with fluids, insulin, and monitoring.

If these symptoms are present, seek immediate medical care.

Severe high blood sugar

Very high blood sugar can also lead to serious problems, especially in older adults.

This condition develops more gradually but can become dangerous.

Symptoms may include:

- extreme thirst
- frequent urination
- dry skin
- weakness
- confusion

This also requires urgent medical attention.

Illness and blood sugar

Even a minor illness can affect blood sugar significantly.

During illness:

- blood sugar may rise

- appetite may decrease
- dehydration may occur

Basic principles include:

- checking blood sugar more frequently
- continuing medications as advised
- drinking fluids
- seeking help if levels remain high

When to seek help immediately

Do not delay medical care if:

- blood sugar is very low and not improving
- there is confusion or unconsciousness
- symptoms of DKA are present
- blood sugar remains very high
- there are signs of dehydration

Early action can prevent serious complications.

Confidence through preparation

At first, these situations may feel frightening.

But with knowledge and preparation, they become manageable.

Knowing what to look for and what to do gives you confidence.

Chapter 9 Summary

- Diabetes emergencies can develop quickly
- Hypoglycemia is common and requires immediate treatment
- Early symptoms include sweating and shakiness
- Severe hypoglycemia can lead to confusion or unconsciousness
- DKA is a serious condition caused by lack of insulin
- Severe high blood sugar can also be dangerous
- Illness can affect blood sugar
- Early recognition and action are essential

Action Plan

- learn the early signs of low and high blood sugar
- keep fast-acting glucose available
- monitor blood sugar regularly
- follow sick-day guidelines during illness
- educate family members about warning signs
- seek medical help promptly when needed
- stay calm and prepared

Looking ahead

Now that we have discussed urgent situations, we turn to one of the most powerful tools in managing diabetes.

In the next chapter, we will focus on diet and nutrition, and how everyday food choices affect blood sugar. Food is something you deal with every single day.

Unlike medications, which you may take once or twice daily, food decisions happen multiple times a day. That is why diet plays such a central role in diabetes care.

The encouraging part is this. You do not need a perfect diet. You need a sensible and sustainable one.

In the next chapter, we will simplify this topic and help you make practical food choices that you can follow comfortably in your daily life.

This is where many patients begin to see real improvement.

Chapter 10

Eating Well with Diabetes: A Simple and Practical Approach

Clearing the confusion about food

If there is one topic that creates the most confusion in diabetes, it is diet.

Almost every patient asks me the same question.

"Doctor, what should I eat?"

They have often heard many different opinions. Some are told to avoid all sugar. Others are advised to follow strict or complicated diets. Many begin to feel that food has suddenly become something to fear.

Let me reassure you at the very beginning.

You do not need a complicated or restrictive diet to manage diabetes well.

You need a clear, balanced, and practical approach that fits into your daily life.

Understanding how food affects blood sugar

To make good decisions, it helps to understand one simple principle.

Carbohydrates are the main nutrients that raise blood sugar.

These include:

- rice, bread, and pasta
- fruits
- milk and yogurt
- sweets and sugary foods

When you eat carbohydrates, they are broken down into glucose and enter the bloodstream.

This is normal and necessary.

The goal is not to eliminate carbohydrates, but to choose wisely and control the amount.

Not all carbohydrates are the same

Some carbohydrates are absorbed quickly and raise blood sugar rapidly.

Others are absorbed more slowly and lead to a gradual rise.

Foods that raise blood sugar quickly include:

- sugary drinks
- sweets and desserts
- refined grains such as white bread

Better choices include:

- whole grains
- vegetables
- legumes
- fruits with natural fiber

These help maintain a more stable blood sugar level.

Portion control: a key concept

Even healthy foods can raise blood sugar if eaten in large amounts.

Portion control is often more important than completely avoiding certain foods.

A simple way to plan meals is the plate method:

- half the plate with non-starchy vegetables
- one quarter with protein
- one quarter with carbohydrates

This approach is easy to follow and works well for most people.

The importance of meal timing

When you eat also matters.

Irregular meals can lead to fluctuations in blood sugar.

Skipping meals may increase the risk of low blood sugar, especially if you are taking medications.

Eating at regular times helps maintain better stability.

Sugary drinks: the easiest change to make

One of the simplest and most effective changes is reducing sugary drinks.

These include:

- soda
- fruit juices
- sweetened tea or coffee
- energy drinks

They raise blood sugar quickly and provide little lasting nutrition.

Replacing them with water or unsweetened beverages can make a significant difference.

A realistic approach to eating

Many patients believe they must follow a strict diet to control diabetes.

That is not necessary.

A good eating plan should be:

- balanced
- flexible
- practical
- sustainable

It should allow you to enjoy food while making better choices most of the time.

Eating outside and social situations

Social meals are part of life.

You do not need to avoid them.

With a little planning, you can manage well:

- choose grilled or baked foods
- control portion sizes
- limit sugary drinks
- avoid overeating

These small adjustments help you stay on track.

Weight and blood sugar

For many patients with type 2 diabetes, weight plays an important role.

Even modest weight loss can improve blood sugar control.

The focus should be on gradual, steady improvement, not extreme dieting.

Avoiding confusion and misinformation

There is a lot of information about diet, and not all of it is reliable.

Some diets promise quick results but are difficult to maintain.

A balanced, evidence-based approach works best.

When in doubt, discuss with your doctor.

A simple way to think about food

Instead of strict rules, think in terms of patterns.

What you eat regularly matters more than occasional choices.

Food should not become a source of stress.

It should remain a normal and enjoyable part of your life.

Chapter 10 Summary

- Diet plays a central role in diabetes management
- Carbohydrates have the greatest effect on blood sugar
- Not all carbohydrates are the same
- Portion control is essential

DIABETES DIET PLAN

EAT MORE

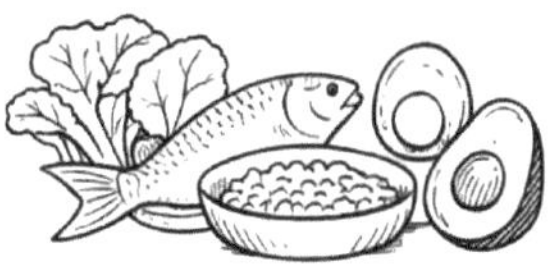

- Vegetables & Greens
- Lean Proteins
- Whole Grains

EAT LESS

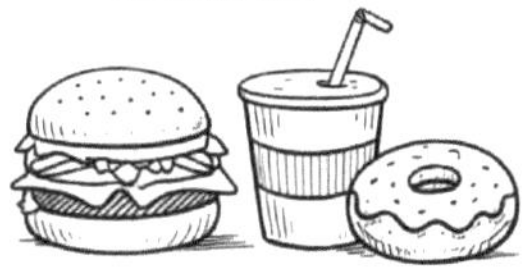

- Sugary Foods
- Refined Carbs
- Fried & Fatty Foods

CONTROL PORTIONS

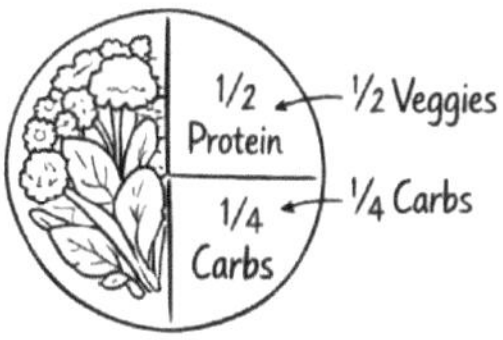

FOCUS ON FIBER

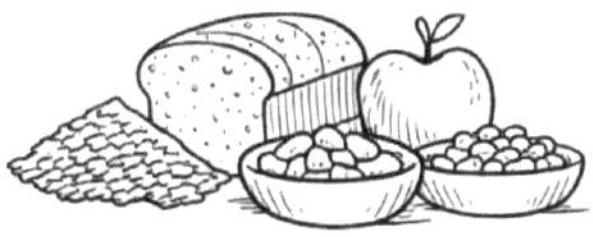

- Whole Grains
- Legumes & Beans
- Fruits & Nuts

STAY HYDRATED

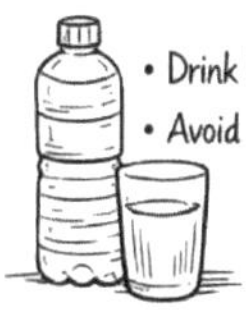

- Drink Plenty of Water
- Avoid Sugary Drinks

EXERCISE REGULARLY

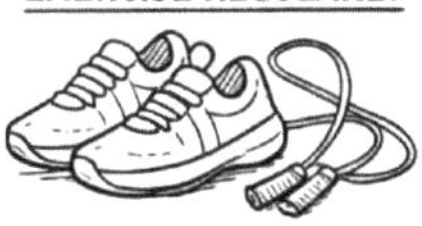

- 30 min Activity Daily
- Walk, Jog, or Bike

MONITOR BLOOD SUGAR

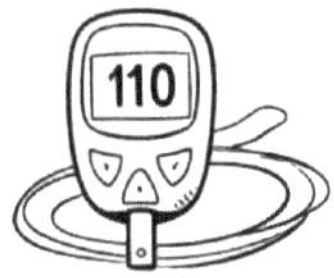

- Check Levels Regularly
- Track Your Results

- Regular meal timing helps maintain stability
- Sugary drinks significantly raise blood sugar
- A balanced and sustainable diet is most effective
- Small, consistent changes lead to lasting benefits

Action Plan

- pay attention to the type and amount of carbohydrates
- use the plate method for meal planning
- reduce or avoid sugary drinks
- eat meals at regular times
- make gradual, sustainable changes
- monitor how food affects your blood sugar
- seek guidance when needed

Looking ahead

Diet is one of the most powerful tools in managing diabetes.

But it is only one part of the overall plan.

In the next chapter, we will focus on lifestyle, including exercise, sleep, stress, and daily habits, and how they influence blood sugar control.

This is where daily routine becomes treatment.

Chapter 11

Lifestyle as Treatment: Movement, Sleep, Stress, and Daily Habits

The treatment you live every day

When people think about treating diabetes, they often think about medications.

But in real life, the most powerful treatment happens outside the clinic.

It happens in your daily routine.

How much you move. How well you sleep. How you handle stress. How regular your habits are.

These factors influence your blood sugar every day, often more than you realize.

The encouraging part is this.

These are areas where you have direct control.

Why movement matters so much

Physical activity is one of the most effective ways to improve blood sugar control.

When you move, your muscles use glucose for energy. This helps lower blood sugar levels.

Over time, regular activity also improves how your body responds to insulin.

This means your body uses glucose more efficiently.

You do not need intense exercise.

Simple activities such as:

- walking
- cycling
- swimming
- light home exercises

can make a real difference.

Building a routine you can follow

Patients often ask, "How much exercise do I need?"

A practical goal is to stay active on most days.

Even 20 to 30 minutes of moderate activity, such as brisk walking, is beneficial.

If you are not used to exercise, start slowly.

A short walk is a good beginning.

What matters most is consistency.

Strength and flexibility

In addition to walking or similar activities, strength exercises are important.

Muscle helps the body use glucose more effectively.

Flexibility exercises help maintain mobility and reduce stiffness.

You do not need a gym.

Simple exercises at home can be enough.

Weight and its role

For many people with type 2 diabetes, excess weight contributes to insulin resistance.

Even modest weight loss can improve blood sugar control.

The goal is steady and sustainable change.

Quick fixes rarely last.

The importance of sleep

Sleep is often overlooked, but it has a direct effect on blood sugar.

Poor sleep can:

- increase insulin resistance
- affect appetite
- increase stress

Patients who do not sleep well often find it harder to control their diabetes.

A regular sleep routine supports better health.

Stress and blood sugar

Stress affects both the body and behavior.

Stress hormones can raise blood sugar.

At the same time, stress may lead to:

- irregular eating
- reduced activity
- poor sleep

This combination can make control more difficult.

Simple ways to manage stress

You do not need complicated techniques.

Simple approaches can help:

- taking short breaks during the day
- slow, steady breathing

- spending time with family
- doing activities you enjoy

Even small changes can make a difference.

Building habits that last

Lifestyle is not about one good day.

It is about repeated habits.

Healthy habits include:

- regular activity
- balanced meals
- consistent sleep
- taking medications as prescribed
- monitoring blood sugar

These do not need to be perfect.

They need to be consistent.

Habits that work against you

Some habits make diabetes harder to manage:

- smoking
- excessive alcohol
- prolonged inactivity

- irregular daily routines

Reducing these has a clear benefit.

Progress, not perfection

This is one of the most important ideas in diabetes care.

You do not need to be perfect.

Trying to change everything at once often leads to frustration.

Instead, focus on small improvements.

A short walk. A better meal. A consistent routine.

These small steps, repeated daily, create lasting results.

Creating a sustainable lifestyle

The goal is not a short-term effort.

It is a way of living.

There will be days when things do not go as planned.

That is normal.

What matters is returning to your routine and continuing forward.

Chapter 11 Summary

- Lifestyle plays a central role in diabetes management
- Physical activity improves blood sugar control

- Regular exercise does not need to be intense
- Weight management helps reduce insulin resistance
- Sleep and stress affect blood sugar significantly
- Healthy habits support long-term health
- Avoiding smoking and excess alcohol is important
- Consistency matters more than perfection

Action Plan

- begin regular physical activity, even short walks
- aim for consistent, good-quality sleep
- practice simple stress management
- work toward gradual weight improvement
- build daily habits
- reduce smoking and alcohol
- stay patient and consistent

Looking ahead

Lifestyle changes form the foundation of diabetes care.

However, many patients also need medications.

In the next chapter, we will discuss oral diabetes medicines, how they work, and how to use them safely.

This will help you approach treatment with clarity and confidence.

Chapter 12

Oral Diabetes Medicines: Clear, Practical Choices

When lifestyle needs support

Many patients begin with diet and lifestyle changes.

For some, especially early on, this may be enough.

For many others, it is not.

This is not a failure.

It reflects how diabetes changes over time. The body may produce less insulin, or insulin may not work as well as it should. When that happens, medications help restore balance.

Think of medicines as support for your body, not a replacement for your efforts.

Why medications are used

Diabetes is not caused by a single problem.

Several processes are involved:

- the liver may produce too much glucose
- the body may not respond well to insulin
- the pancreas may not produce enough insulin

Different medications target these different problems.

They may:

- improve insulin sensitivity
- increase insulin release
- reduce glucose production
- slow glucose absorption

Using the right combination improves control.

Metformin: the usual starting point

For most patients with type 2 diabetes, treatment begins with metformin.

It works by:

- reducing glucose production in the liver
- improving the body's response to insulin

It has been used for many years and is generally safe.

Some patients notice mild stomach discomfort at the beginning, but this usually improves with time or dose adjustment.

It has a low risk of causing low blood sugar when used alone.

Other commonly used medicines

There are several other types of oral medications.

Some help the pancreas release more insulin.

Others help the body use insulin more effectively.

Some reduce the amount of glucose absorbed from food.

Newer medications have additional benefits:

- support weight control
- reduce cardiovascular risk
- help protect kidney function

Your doctor will choose based on your individual needs.

Why more than one medication may be needed

Over time, many patients need more than one medication.

This does not mean your condition is suddenly worsening.

It reflects the progressive nature of diabetes.

Using different medications together often works better than increasing the dose of a single drug.

Benefits and possible side effects

All medications have benefits and potential side effects.

Benefits include:

- better blood sugar control
- reduced risk of complications
- improved energy and well-being

Possible side effects vary depending on the drug and may include:

- stomach discomfort
- risk of low blood sugar with certain medicines
- weight changes

Most side effects are manageable with proper guidance.

Taking medications regularly

Medications only work when taken consistently.

Common challenges include:

- forgetting doses
- stopping when you feel better
- concern about side effects

Consistency is essential.

A simple routine helps maintain stable control.

Addressing common concerns

Many patients hesitate to start medication.

Some feel it means they have failed.

Others worry about long-term use.

It is important to understand:

Medications are tools.

They help the body function more effectively and prevent complications.

Starting them at the right time protects your health.

Monitoring while on medication

Regular monitoring is important when taking medications.

This includes:

- checking blood sugar
- periodic blood tests

Monitoring ensures that treatment is working and remains safe.

Individualized treatment

There is no single plan that works for everyone.

Treatment depends on:

- age

- duration of diabetes
- other health conditions
- lifestyle
- risk of low blood sugar

This individualized approach leads to better results.

Medications as part of the bigger picture

Medications are only one part of diabetes care.

They work best when combined with:

- balanced diet
- regular activity
- good sleep
- ongoing monitoring

A practical perspective

The goal is not to avoid medication.

The goal is to achieve good control and protect long-term health.

Chapter 12 Summary

- Many patients need medications in addition to lifestyle changes

Types of Medicines in Diabetes

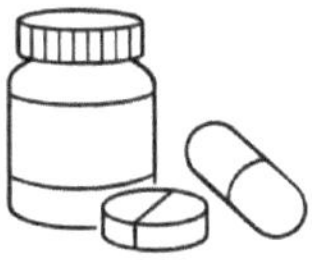

ORAL MEDICATIONS

Pills that help lower blood sugar levels.

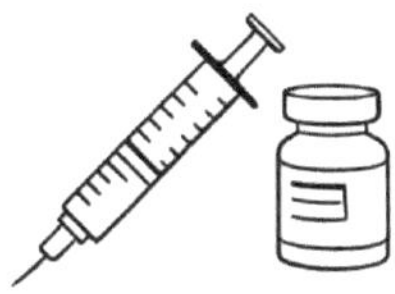

INSULIN THERAPY

Insulin injections to manage blood sugar.

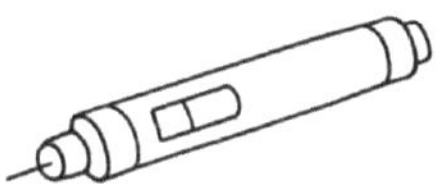

GLP-1 RECEPTOR AGONISTS

Injectable meds that aid in blood sugar control.

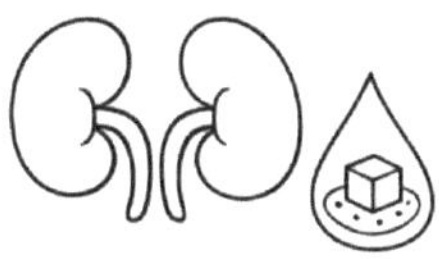

SGLT2 INHIBITORS

Helps kidneys remove excess sugar.

- Oral medicines work in different ways
- Metformin is usually the first choice
- Combination therapy is common
- Medications have benefits and possible side effects
- Consistent use is essential
- Treatment should be individualized

Action Plan

- take medications as prescribed
- do not stop medications without consulting your doctor
- monitor blood sugar regularly
- report side effects promptly
- understand the purpose of each medication
- combine medication with healthy habits

Looking ahead

Oral medications are an important part of diabetes care.

However, many patients eventually need insulin.

In the next chapter, we will discuss insulin therapy, when it is needed, and how to use it safely and confidently.

This will help remove fear and build confidence.

Chapter 13

Insulin Made Simple: When You Need It and How to Use It Well

Moving past the hesitation

There is a moment I have seen many times in my practice.

We discuss treatment, and I mention insulin. The room becomes quiet. The patient looks concerned.

“Doctor, does this mean my diabetes has become serious?”

It is a natural reaction.

Let me reassure you clearly.

Insulin is not a sign of failure. It is a natural hormone your body needs. When your body cannot produce enough, we simply replace what is missing.

When used properly, insulin is one of the most effective and reliable treatments in diabetes care.

What insulin actually does

Insulin plays a central role in how your body uses glucose.

It helps glucose move from the bloodstream into the cells, where it is used for energy.

It also:

- reduces glucose production by the liver
- helps store excess glucose for later use

Without enough insulin, glucose builds up in the blood instead of being used.

Insulin therapy helps restore this balance.

When insulin becomes necessary

Insulin is essential in type 1 diabetes.

In type 2 diabetes, it may be needed:

- when oral medications are not enough
- during illness or physical stress
- during pregnancy
- when the pancreas produces less insulin over time

In some cases, insulin is used temporarily. In others, it becomes part of long-term care.

Common concerns and how to address them

Patients often worry about:

- injections
- managing doses
- risk of low blood sugar
- long-term use

These concerns are understandable.

But modern insulin therapy is much simpler than many people expect. With proper guidance, most patients learn quickly and become comfortable.

How insulin is given

Insulin is usually given as a small injection under the skin.

Common sites include:

- abdomen
- thighs
- upper arms

The needles used today are very fine. Most patients find the process much easier than they expected.

Insulin pens have made administration simple and convenient.

Using insulin safely

Safe use of insulin involves a few key steps:

- taking the correct dose
- timing it properly with meals or routine
- monitoring blood sugar
- storing insulin correctly

At first, this may seem like a lot.

With practice, it becomes part of your daily routine.

Preventing low blood sugar

The most important concern with insulin is low blood sugar.

It may occur if:

- too much insulin is taken
- meals are delayed or skipped
- physical activity increases without adjustment

Balancing insulin, food, and activity is essential.

Regular monitoring helps you understand how your body responds.

Adjusting to daily life

Starting insulin often requires some adjustments.

You may need to:

- check your blood sugar more often
- be mindful of meal timing
- plan for physical activity

At first, this may feel unfamiliar.

Over time, it becomes manageable and routine.

Benefits of insulin therapy

Insulin offers clear benefits:

- improved blood sugar control
- reduction in symptoms such as fatigue and excessive thirst
- lower risk of complications
- improved overall well-being

Many patients feel better once their blood sugar levels are better controlled.

Working with your doctor

Insulin therapy works best with good communication.

You should feel comfortable discussing:

- your blood sugar readings
- any episodes of low or high blood sugar
- concerns about dosing

Adjustments are often needed and are a normal part of care.

A practical way to think about insulin

Think of insulin as a tool.

It is used when needed to help your body function properly.

The goal is not to avoid insulin.

The goal is to use the right treatment at the right time.

Confidence grows with experience

At first, insulin may feel unfamiliar.

With time, practice, and understanding, it becomes easier.

Many patients who were hesitant at the beginning later feel confident and comfortable using it.

Chapter 13 Summary

- Insulin is a natural hormone that regulates blood sugar
- It is essential in type 1 diabetes and often needed in type 2 diabetes
- Insulin therapy is not a failure
- Modern injection methods are simple and effective
- Safe use requires correct dosing and monitoring
- Low blood sugar is the main risk

INSULIN THERAPY

Types of Insulin

- Rapid-Acting
- Short-Acting
- Intermediate-Acting
- Long-Acting

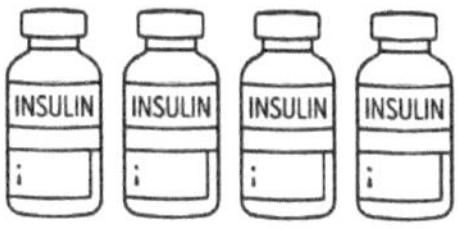

Injection Sites

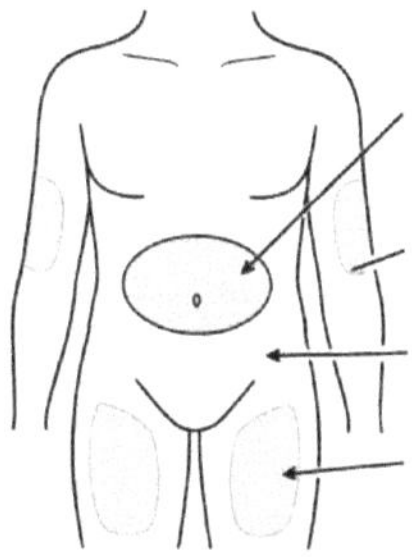

Delivery Methods

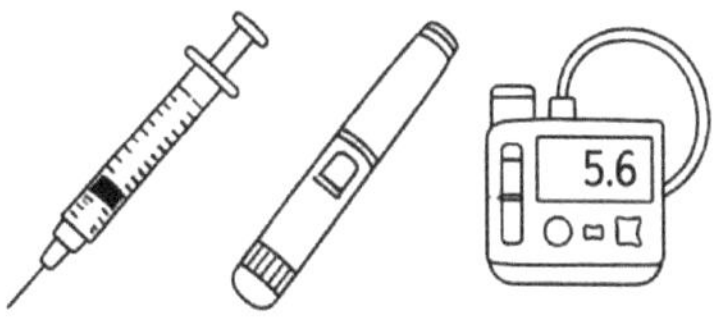

Insulin Syringe Insulin Pen Insulin Pump

Tips for Safe Use

- Store insulin properly (refrigeration may be needed)
- Check expiration dates
- Rotate injection sites
- Use the correct dose
- Follow your healthcare provider's instructions

Benefits of Insulin Therapy

- Controls Blood Sugar
- Reduces Complications
- Improves Energy Levels
- Supports Overall Health

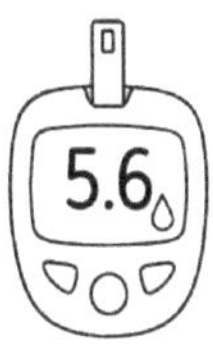

When to Contact Your Healthcare Provider

- Frequent low blood sugar (hypoglycemia)
- Symptoms of high blood sugar (hyperglycemia)
- Unusual symptoms or side effects

- Insulin improves symptoms and reduces complications
- Confidence develops over time

Action Plan

- learn how insulin works
- follow your dosing schedule carefully
- monitor your blood sugar regularly
- recognize signs of low blood sugar
- communicate with your doctor
- focus on consistency and safety

Looking ahead

Now that you understand insulin, the next step is to learn about the different types of insulin and the newer technologies available.

In the next chapter, we will discuss insulin types, inhaled insulin, insulin pumps, and continuous glucose monitoring.

This will help you choose what fits your lifestyle best.

Chapter 14

Types of Insulin and Modern Technology: Choosing What Works for You

From confusion to clarity

At some point, many patients feel overwhelmed.

They hear about different types of insulin, pens, pumps, sensors, and newer technologies.

"Doctor, there are so many options. How do I choose?"

That is a very reasonable question.

The answer is simpler than it seems.

You do not need to understand everything at once. You only need to understand the basics and choose what fits your life.

How the body normally uses insulin

In a healthy body, insulin is released in two ways:

- a steady level throughout the day
- extra amounts after meals

Modern insulin therapy is designed to copy this natural pattern.

That is why there are different types of insulin.

Rapid-acting insulin

Rapid-acting insulin works quickly.

It is taken around mealtime to control the rise in blood sugar after eating.

It begins to act within minutes and lasts for a short time.

This makes it ideal for controlling post-meal blood sugar.

Short-acting insulin

Short-acting insulin also helps control blood sugar after meals, but it works a little more slowly.

It is usually taken before meals.

It is used less frequently now because rapid-acting insulin is more predictable.

Intermediate-acting insulin

This type works more slowly and lasts longer.

It provides background insulin coverage for part of the day or night.

It is sometimes used in combination with other types.

Long-acting insulin

Long-acting insulin provides a steady level of insulin over a full day.

It helps control blood sugar between meals and during sleep.

Many patients take it once daily, sometimes twice.

It forms the foundation of many treatment plans.

Premixed insulin

Premixed insulin combines two types of insulin in one injection.

It can be convenient because it reduces the number of injections.

However, it offers less flexibility in adjusting doses.

It is often suitable for patients with regular meal schedules.

Inhaled insulin

Inhaled insulin is a newer option.

It is taken through the lungs and works quickly, similar to rapid-acting insulin.

It may be useful for some patients who prefer to avoid injections at mealtime.

However, it is not suitable for everyone, especially those with lung conditions.

Ways to deliver insulin

In addition to different types of insulin, there are different ways to deliver it.

Syringes

An older method, still effective but used less often today.

Insulin pens

The most common method. Simple, convenient, and accurate.

Insulin pumps

Small devices that deliver insulin continuously through a thin tube under the skin.

They provide steady background insulin and allow additional doses at mealtime.

Pumps offer flexibility but require training.

Continuous glucose monitoring (CGM)

One of the most important advances in diabetes care is continuous glucose monitoring.

A small sensor placed under the skin measures glucose levels throughout the day and night.

It provides:

- real-time readings
- trends and patterns
- alerts for high or low levels

This information helps you make better decisions in daily life.

Toward automated systems

Some newer systems combine insulin pumps with continuous glucose monitoring.

These systems can adjust insulin delivery automatically based on glucose levels.

They reduce the need for constant manual adjustments.

While not perfect, they make diabetes management easier and more precise.

Choosing what fits your life

Patients often ask which option is best.

There is no single answer.

The right choice depends on:

- your type of diabetes

- your daily routine
- your comfort with technology
- cost and access

The goal is to find a plan that is effective and practical.

Keeping it simple

More advanced technology is not always necessary.

Some patients do very well with simple treatment plans.

Others benefit from more advanced systems.

The key is to choose what you can use consistently.

Learning step by step

At first, these options may seem complicated.

With time and guidance, they become easier to understand.

You do not need to master everything at once.

Confidence grows gradually.

Chapter 14 Summary

- Different types of insulin mimic the body's natural pattern
- Rapid-acting insulin controls blood sugar after meals
- Long-acting insulin provides steady background control

- Premixed insulin offers convenience but less flexibility
- Inhaled insulin is an option for selected patients
- Insulin can be delivered through pens, syringes, or pumps
- CGM provides real-time glucose information
- Treatment should be individualized

Action Plan

- understand the type of insulin you are using
- follow your dosing schedule carefully
- discuss delivery options with your doctor
- consider CGM if appropriate
- keep your treatment plan simple
- monitor your blood sugar regularly

Looking ahead

So far, we have focused on the medical and practical aspects of diabetes.

In the next chapter, we will discuss the emotional and social side of living with diabetes.

This is an important part of long-term success.

Chapter 15

The Emotional and Social Side of Diabetes: Living Beyond the Numbers

The part that is often left unspoken

So far, we have talked about tests, medications, food, and daily routines.

All of these are important.

But there is another side of diabetes that is just as real.

How you feel.

How you think about your condition.

How it affects your daily life, your family, and your relationships.

Over the years, I have seen many patients manage their blood sugar quite well, yet quietly struggle with worry, frustration, or fatigue related to their condition.

This chapter is about that side of the journey.

The emotional impact of diagnosis

When someone is first told they have diabetes, the reaction is rarely simple.

Some feel shocked.

Some feel worried about the future.

Some feel guilty.

I remember a patient who sat quietly for a few moments after hearing the diagnosis and then said, "I always thought this would not happen to me."

That reaction is very human.

It takes time to understand, accept, and adjust.

What matters is not the initial reaction, but how you move forward from there.

Living with a condition that requires attention

Diabetes is not something you deal with once and forget.

It requires ongoing attention.

Patients often describe a feeling of always having to think about it.

What to eat. When to eat. Medications. Monitoring.

Over time, this can feel tiring.

This is sometimes called burnout.

It is not a weakness. It is a natural response to managing a long-term condition.

Stress and its effect on blood sugar

Stress affects both the body and behavior.

When you are under stress, certain hormones are released that can raise blood sugar.

At the same time, stress may lead to:

- irregular eating
- reduced physical activity
- poor sleep

This creates a cycle that can make diabetes harder to manage.

Family and relationships

Diabetes often affects more than one person.

It can influence family routines, meals, and social activities.

Some patients feel different or restricted, especially during gatherings.

Family members may want to help but may not always know how.

Open communication makes a difference.

When your family understands your condition, they can support you in a meaningful way.

Social situations and food

Food is often central to social life.

Celebrations, family events, and gatherings can feel challenging.

You do not need to avoid these situations.

Instead:

- make thoughtful choices
- watch portion sizes
- plan ahead

With time, these adjustments become natural.

Work, travel, and daily routine

Diabetes must fit into your life, not the other way around.

At work, you may need to:

- plan meals
- monitor blood sugar
- take medications

During travel, some preparation helps.

Carrying medications and maintaining a basic routine makes things easier.

When emotional health needs attention

Sometimes, emotional challenges go beyond normal adjustment.

You may notice:

- persistent sadness
- anxiety
- lack of motivation
- feeling overwhelmed

If this happens, it is important to seek help.

Talking to a healthcare provider or counselor can make a meaningful difference.

Emotional health is part of overall health.

Building a support system

You do not have to manage diabetes alone.

Support can come from:

- family
- friends
- healthcare providers
- support groups

Sharing your experience often reduces stress and makes the journey easier.

Finding balance

Some patients become very strict and anxious about every detail.

Others feel discouraged and stop trying.

Neither approach works well.

A balanced approach is more effective.

Aim for consistency rather than perfection.

Living a full life

One of the most important messages I share with my patients is this.

Diabetes should not prevent you from living your life.

With proper management, you can continue to:

- work
- travel
- enjoy family life
- pursue your interests

The goal is not only to control blood sugar, but to maintain a good quality of life.

Confidence grows over time

As you gain experience, something important happens.

You begin to feel more confident.

You understand your body better. You know how to respond. You feel less uncertain.

This confidence develops gradually, but it is real.

Chapter 15 Summary

- Diabetes affects emotional and social life as well as physical health
- Patients may experience stress, worry, or burnout
- Family and social situations can present challenges
- Communication and planning help manage these situations
- Emotional health is an important part of care
- Support systems improve coping and confidence
- Balance is more effective than perfection
- Patients can live full and active lives

Action Plan

- acknowledge your feelings without judgment
- communicate openly with family and friends
- plan for social situations
- maintain a balanced approach
- seek help if you feel overwhelmed
- build a support system

- focus on living well

Looking ahead

We have now covered the medical, practical, and emotional aspects of diabetes.

In the final chapter, we will bring everything together into a clear and practical plan for long-term living.

We will focus on how to stay consistent, confident, and in control over time.

Chapter 16

Living Well for the Long Term: A Simple Plan That Works

Bringing everything together

If you have read this far, you have already taken an important step.

You have moved from uncertainty toward understanding. From scattered information toward a clearer picture of diabetes and how to manage it.

Now the question becomes practical.

How do you live with this, day after day, year after year, without feeling overwhelmed?

The answer is simpler than most people expect.

What really matters over time

In my years of practice, I have seen a consistent pattern.

The patients who do well are not those who try to do everything perfectly.

They are the ones who stay steady.

They:

- follow a routine
- make sensible choices most of the time
- stay engaged in their care
- adjust when needed

It is this steady approach that leads to good long-term results.

The core pillars of care

By now, you have seen that diabetes management rests on a few key areas:

- understanding your condition
- eating in a balanced way
- staying physically active
- taking medications when needed
- monitoring blood sugar
- maintaining regular follow-up

You do not need to master all of these at once.

You need to work on them consistently.

Keeping it practical in daily life

Patients often feel overwhelmed when thinking about long-term care.

I suggest a simpler approach.

Focus on today.

- make a better food choice today
- take a short walk today
- take your medication today
- check your blood sugar as advised

These small actions, repeated daily, create long-term results.

Adapting as life changes

Life is not static.

Your schedule, your health, your responsibilities, all change over time.

Your diabetes management should adapt as well.

There will be times when control is better and times when it becomes more challenging.

This is normal.

What matters is staying involved and making adjustments when needed.

Preventing complications

One of the main goals of diabetes care is to prevent complications.

As you have learned, many complications develop slowly and can often be prevented.

This depends on:

- steady blood sugar control
- healthy habits
- regular medical care
- timely adjustments in treatment

Even moderate improvement can make a meaningful difference.

Using available tools wisely

Modern diabetes care offers many tools:

- medications
- insulin
- monitoring devices
- educational resources

You do not need to use everything.

Use what fits your needs.

The goal is to make your care easier and more effective.

Staying informed without feeling overwhelmed

It is helpful to stay informed about your condition.

But too much information can sometimes feel overwhelming.

Focus on clear and reliable guidance.

Learn step by step.

Ask questions when needed.

A balanced mindset

Managing diabetes is not about strict control at every moment.

It is about balance.

There will be good days and less ideal days.

Do not be discouraged.

Return to your routine and continue.

Living your life fully

Diabetes is one part of your life.

It is not your entire life.

With proper management, you can continue to:

- work

- travel
- enjoy your family
- pursue your interests

The goal is not only control, but a good quality of life.

One simple message

If there is one message I would like you to remember, it is this.

Do not try to manage diabetes for the rest of your life all at once.

Focus on today.

Make one good decision today.

Then do the same tomorrow.

Confidence grows with time

Over time, something important happens.

You begin to feel more confident.

You understand your body better. You know how to respond. You feel less uncertain.

This confidence builds gradually.

Chapter 16 Summary

- Long-term success depends on consistency

- Diabetes management rests on key pillars
- Small daily actions create lasting results
- Management should adapt over time
- Many complications can be prevented
- Use available tools as needed
- Balance is more important than perfection
- Diabetes should not limit your life

Action Plan

- focus on simple, consistent daily habits
- follow your treatment plan
- stay active and eat in a balanced way
- attend regular follow-up
- adjust your plan when needed
- stay positive and realistic
- continue learning

Conclusion

A Steady Path Forward

When I reflect on my years in medicine, one lesson stands out clearly.

The patients who do well are not the ones who try to do everything

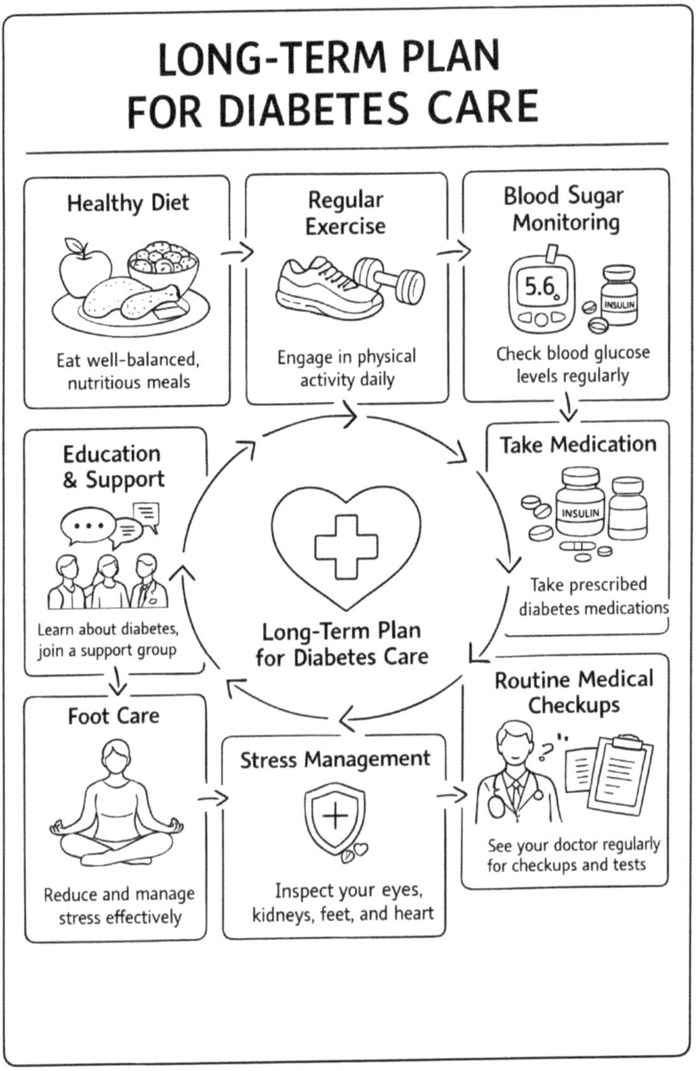
LONG-TERM PLAN
FOR DIABETES CARE
Healthy Diet
Eat well-balanced, nutritious meals
Regular Exercise
Engage in physical activity daily
Blood Sugar Monitoring
5.6
INSULIN
Check blood glucose levels regularly
Take Medication
INSULIN
Take prescribed diabetes medications
Routine Medical Checkups
See your doctor regularly for checkups and tests
Stress Management
Inspect your eyes, kidneys, feet, and heart
Foot Care
Reduce and manage stress effectively
Education & Support
Learn about diabetes, join a support group
Long-Term Plan for Diabetes Care

perfectly.

They are the ones who stay steady.

They learn. They adjust. They continue.

If you take one message from this book, let it be this.

Diabetes is manageable.

Not in a dramatic or complicated way, but in a steady, practical way.

You do not need to change everything at once.

You need to take one step at a time.

A better meal. A short walk. Taking your medication regularly. Paying attention to your health.

These simple actions, repeated day after day, have a powerful effect.

There will be challenges. That is part of any long-term condition.

But with understanding, consistency, and support, you can move forward with confidence.

You can live well with diabetes.

Chapter 17

Frequently Asked Questions and Common Myths About Diabetes

Clearing confusion, building confidence

Over the years, I have noticed that patients with diabetes often carry many doubts.

Some come from half-correct information.

Some from the internet.

Some from well-meaning friends and family.

Many of these beliefs create unnecessary fear or confusion.

In this chapter, I will address some of the most common questions and myths in a simple and practical way.

"Did I get diabetes because I ate too much sugar?"

This is one of the most common concerns.

The answer is not so simple.

Eating excess sugar over time can contribute to weight gain, and weight gain can increase the risk of type 2 diabetes.

But diabetes is not caused by sugar alone.

Genetics, lifestyle, body weight, and how your body handles insulin all play a role.

So, it is not a single cause.

And it is certainly not something to feel guilty about.

"Can diabetes be completely cured?"

At present, diabetes is generally a long-term condition.

In some people, especially early in type 2 diabetes, blood sugar can return to near normal levels with weight loss and lifestyle changes.

This is often called remission.

But the underlying tendency remains.

That is why ongoing care and attention are still important.

"Do I have to stop eating sweets completely?"

No.

You do not have to completely eliminate sweets.

What matters is moderation and balance.

Occasional sweets, in small amounts and as part of a balanced meal, can be included.

The problem is not a single dessert. It is frequent excess.

"If I start medication, will I need it forever?"

Not always.

Some patients may reduce or adjust medications with lifestyle improvement.

Others may need medications long term.

This depends on how the body responds over time.

Taking medication when needed is a way to protect your health, not a sign of failure.

"Is insulin a last option?"

Many people believe insulin is used only when everything else fails.

This is not correct.

Insulin is simply another treatment option.

It is used when the body needs it.

In some situations, it is used temporarily. In others, it is part of long-term care.

It is a tool, not a punishment.

"Can I manage diabetes with diet alone?"

Some people can, especially early in the condition.

But many need medications along with diet and lifestyle.

The goal is good control, not avoiding treatment.

"Are natural remedies enough?"

Many natural approaches may support general health.

But they are usually not enough by themselves to control diabetes.

Relying only on unproven remedies can delay proper treatment.

It is always better to use evidence-based treatment and discuss any supplements with your doctor.

"Why is my blood sugar high even when I am careful?"

This can be frustrating.

Blood sugar is influenced by many factors:

- stress
- illness
- sleep
- medications

- natural body changes

Even when you are careful, variations can occur.

Look at patterns over time rather than a single reading.

"Can I live a normal life with diabetes?"

Yes.

This is one of the most important truths.

With proper management, you can:

- work
- travel
- enjoy food
- spend time with family
- live actively

Diabetes requires attention, but it does not take away your ability to live fully.

"Is diabetes always progressive?"

Diabetes can change over time.

In many people, it does progress gradually.

But good control can slow this process significantly.

Some patients maintain stable control for many years.

“Should I be afraid of complications?”

Fear does not help.

Awareness does.

Complications are not inevitable.

They depend largely on how diabetes is managed over time.

With steady care, the risk can be reduced.

A simple way to think about all this

When you hear something about diabetes, ask yourself:

- Is this based on reliable information?
- Does it make sense medically?
- Should I confirm this with my doctor?

This approach helps you avoid confusion.

Confidence comes from clarity

As your understanding improves, many doubts begin to fade.

You feel less anxious.

You feel more in control.

That confidence is an important part of living well with diabetes.

Chapter 17 Summary

- Many beliefs about diabetes are based on incomplete or incorrect information
- Diabetes is caused by multiple factors, not just sugar
- It is a long-term condition but can be well managed
- Medications and insulin are tools, not failures
- Diet and lifestyle are important but may not be enough alone
- Natural remedies should not replace medical treatment
- Blood sugar varies for many reasons
- Patients can live full and active lives with diabetes

Action Plan

- question common myths and seek reliable information
- avoid self-blame
- follow evidence-based treatment
- discuss doubts with your doctor
- focus on long-term consistency
- build confidence through understanding

Appendix A

A Simple Daily Diabetes Checklist

Living well with diabetes does not require complicated steps.

In my experience, patients who do well are those who follow a few simple habits every day, consistently and calmly.

You do not need to do everything perfectly. You need to do the important things regularly.

Here is a simple checklist you can follow.

Every Day

- Take your medications as prescribed
- Eat balanced meals at regular times
- Stay physically active, even a short walk helps
- Monitor your blood sugar as advised
- Drink enough water

- Get adequate sleep
- Check your feet for cuts, redness, or swelling

Every Week

- Review your blood sugar readings
- Notice patterns rather than single numbers
- Check your weight if advised
- Plan your meals for the coming days

A simple reminder

If you feel overwhelmed, come back to this.

Focus on today.

Do the basic things well.

That is enough.

Appendix B

Warning Signs You Should Not Ignore

Most of diabetes develops slowly.

But some symptoms require attention.

Do not ignore these warning signs. Acting early can prevent serious problems.

Contact your doctor if you notice:

- persistent high blood sugar readings
- frequent episodes of low blood sugar
- increasing fatigue without clear reason
- blurred or changing vision
- numbness, tingling, or burning in hands or feet
- wounds that are not healing

- swelling in feet or legs

Seek urgent medical care if you have:

- severe weakness or confusion
- chest discomfort or pressure
- sudden difficulty speaking or understanding
- weakness on one side of the body
- severe vomiting or dehydration
- very high or very low blood sugar not improving

A simple way to think about it

If something feels unusual, persistent, or worsening, do not ignore it.

It is always better to check early than to wait.

Appendix C

A Practical Weekly Plan for Living Well with Diabetes

Many patients ask for a simple structure.

Not a strict schedule, but a practical guide.

Here is one you can follow and adjust based on your lifestyle.

Daily Routine

Morning

- Take medications as prescribed
- Eat a balanced breakfast
- Check blood sugar if advised

Daytime

- Stay active, walking, light exercise, or daily movement

- Eat balanced meals at regular times
- Stay hydrated

Evening

- Eat a moderate dinner
- Take medications if prescribed
- Light activity after meals can help

Night

- Maintain a regular sleep schedule

Weekly Focus

Physical Activity

- Aim for activity on most days
- Include walking and light strength exercises

Food Planning

- Plan meals ahead
- Avoid last-minute unhealthy choices

Monitoring

- Review blood sugar trends
- Notice what affects your readings

Health Check

- Pay attention to feet, skin, and general well-being

A realistic approach

This plan is not meant to be strict.

Life will not always follow a schedule.

That is normal.

Return to your routine the next day and continue.

Consistency over time matters far more than any single day.

Thank You and Please Review the Book

Thank you for taking the time to read this book. I sincerely hope it has helped you understand your health a little more clearly and has given you practical, everyday steps you can follow with confidence. If you found this book helpful, **I would truly appreciate it if you could leave a brief and honest review.** Even a few lines sharing your experience can make a meaningful difference. Your feedback helps other readers find reliable, trustworthy health information and supports them in making better decisions for themselves and their families.

Warm regards,

Dr Prabhat Das

Continue your Healthcare Journey

Good health is a journey, not a single step. It is not achieved in one day or with one book. That is why I created the **"Better Health with Dr Das"** series, with each book addressing a different common condition. If you would like easy, practical guidance on other everyday health concerns, you may wish to explore the rest of books in this series.

Books in this series:

- A Doctor's Easy Guide to Understanding & Managing **OBESITY**.

- A Doctor's Easy Guide to Understanding & Managing **HIGH BLOOD PRESSURE**.

- Doctor, What **DIET** Is Best for Me?

- Doctor, Why Can't I **Lose Weight?**

(a Doctor's Guide to safe & Sustainable Weight Loss)

- A Doctor's Easy Guide to **GLP-1 for Obesity**

- A Doctor's Guide to Living Well With **DIABETES**

• A Doctor's Guide to Understanding & Managing **HIGH CHOLESTEROL**

• A Doctor's Guide to Understanding & **Managing THYROID DISEASES**

9 781971 672359

Printed by Libri Plureos GmbH in Hamburg,
Germany